MW00937275

Raising Ali

THE BFF SERIES: BRAVE, FEARLESS, AND FREE LIVING

Raising *Ali*

NICOLE K. MONTEZ

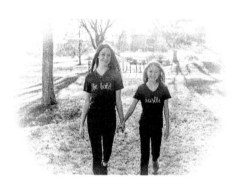

To Ali and Isi,
my ultimate gift is being your mom.
Thank you for giving me purpose.

CONTENTS

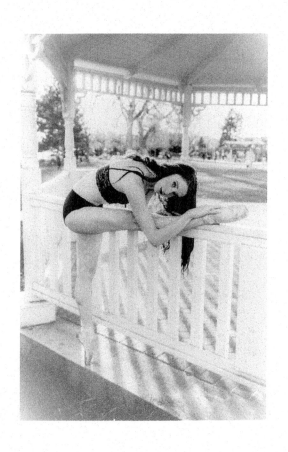

"To be brave and fearless is standing up to your problems and not running away from them, taking care of yourself; staying strong."
-Ali

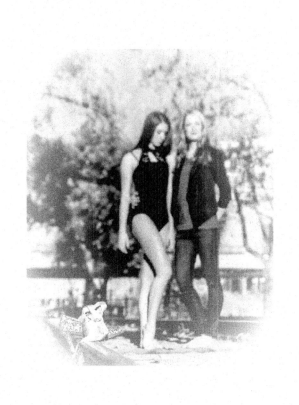

BFF SERIES INTRODUCTION

THE IDEA OF 'THE BFF LIFE' WAS BORN from a deep desire to empower women and moms everywhere to live a life of courage, faith, and freedom. So often we hear or use the phrase 'BFF'. Someone may proclaim "She's my BFF!" meaning her favorite friend, her closest best friend forever. What if there was another way to describe your best friend? What if we were each our very own BFF? Living a purposeful, wholehearted, brave, fearless and free life? Brave, to have bold courage in spite of anything you may face. Fearless, to have faith you will always be ok, and no matter what comes up it is all happening for the greater good. Free, to live a life authentically you, without perfection and the labels and expectations from others.

In this first book of the series, I'm grateful to share my first BFF journey as a mother living with my daughter's diagnosis. A diagnosis that helped me get off the floor of pain, look perfectionism in the face, and find my own journey of living brave, fearless and free. My wish is that this series will help you too find your own personal BFF journey. In this first book, I'm grateful to share with you my first BFF journey as a mother living with my daughter's diagnosis. A diagnosis that helped me get off the floor of pain, and find my own journey of living brave, fearless and free. My wish is that this series will help you too find your own personal BFF journey.

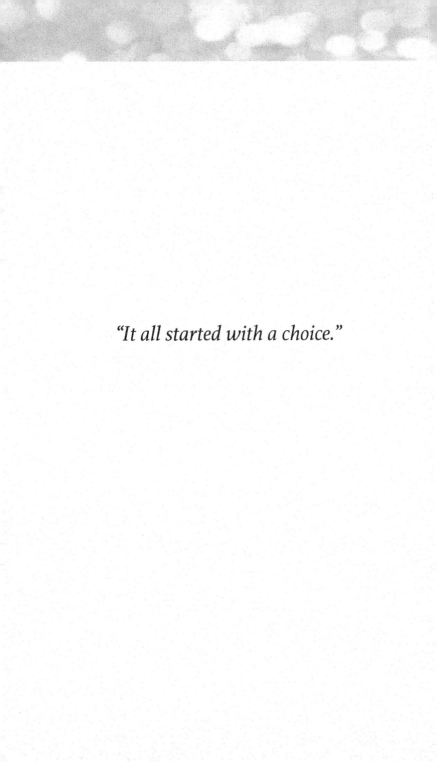

"It all started with a choice."

BLESSED

I WAS ON THE FLOOR. USUALLY THIS occurs only after a fall, or the process of digging under the bed. But this time was different. This was on the floor in unbearable pain. Pain so strong you don't know how you will actually stand up again, or even if you want to. You know if you stand up everything is now different. Life has changed. The game changed. And none of it was part of the plan.

My daughter Ali has cystic fibrosis. Cystic Fibrosis, or CF as it's commonly referred to, is a genetic disease that causes severe damage to the lungs and digestive system and is often fatal. While it's a fairly well-known disease, there are only about 70,000 people living with CF in the entire world, with 1000 new cases diagnosed every year.

Through our journey I've learned that a diagnosis is not a destiny. It's not what defines us. What breaks your heart can lead you to your true purpose. From a wound comes lessons.

Since Ali's diagnosis she's grown to be an amazing young woman. I have been able to start and grow more than one multi-million dollar business as a stay-at-home mom with little to no experience. But it all started with a choice. One decision to get up off the floor and begin my first BFF journey.

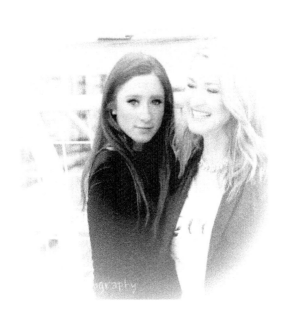

*"Little girls with dreams,
become women with vision."*

ULTIMATE DREAMS

AS FAR BACK AS I CAN REMEMBER I always had a plan. I dreamt about being the CEO of a company. At 3 years old while little girls would push around their dolls in a baby stroller, I was the girl who would push around her books, piles of books. I wanted to be smart. I loved how the books felt, smelled, and the feel of them in my tiny hands. I wanted to be a boss (to be honest I've always been called a little bit 'bossy'), a true business woman one day. Have you ever made a plan for your life? As little girls we laid on our beds and stared at the ceiling dreaming big dreams for ourselves and our grown up lives. We giggled and told our friends of our plans. Innocent plans and we could do anything, be anything, and have anything we wanted. Some girls dreamed of fancy weddings, others wanted to be teachers, some dreamt of being mommies. I was going to be successful and take over corporate America. Even back then as I pushed my stroller down the block, being a mother someday just wasn't something I thought about. It wasn't that I didn't want to, I just didn't think about it.

All went according to plan and after high school I earned a business degree and got a job straight out of college and began working in the recruiting industry. I worked closely with my bosses and studied my mentors. I loved the idea, and the feel of independence and accomplishment in climbing the corporate ladder. It was fascinating to me. When I was 23 I received my 3rd promotion and was offered my dream position. Dan and I had dated a few years and got engaged and began planning our big wedding.

Life was going just according to plan. The same plan I had as a little girl with her stroller of books. I had so many dreams of what the future would look like.

"This wasn't at all part of my plan."

LIFE-CHANGING MOMENT

I STILL REMEMBER THE DAY I FOUND out I was pregnant. It wasn't really the fairytale way I imagined it would be, after all our wedding was just 6 weeks away. There wasn't the story of new wedded bliss and the anticipation and decision of planning a family. Out of nowhere I was quickly learning life wasn't going to happen according to my plan. It was a chilly September day and a normal, but busy day at the office. By mid-morning I was starving so when lunch finally came my office partner and I ran across the street craving McDonald's, and until then it never dawned on me it had been awhile since I remember having my last period.

Just to confirm the 'there is no way I am pregnant' thought, the 'I am not even married yet worry', we stopped by the store for a pregnancy test. It was all quite surreal. In the middle of a workday, unemotional and dressed in my suit and heels, here I was running down the aisle of a grocery store to purchase a quick test and rush back. I wanted to hurry up and move on. Up until then with life I was always on to the next thing. That was the business life. The world of solving problems, finding solutions and always quickly moving forward.

Arriving at the office I nonchalantly made my way to the bathroom and hurried into a stall. I certainly couldn't let anyone to see me. I couldn't really feel anything. We are just simply ruling this out. As I held the white stick I calmly waited for just the one line to come up meaning not pregnant. Reading the box, the test was supposed to take up to 5 minutes, but in less than a minute one line appeared in the little clear window, and just as quickly another darker line appeared next to it. I grabbed the box as surely, I confused the lines and results. Nope I wasn't confused, two lines definitely equals pregnant.

No way. What? How could this be? I have dreams and goals! I had it all mapped out and none of them included becoming a mom anytime soon.

I quickly put the test in my pocket, hid the shock on my face and left the bathroom in utter disbelief. Emotionless with game face on, but inside I was terrified.

Right away I struggled with what to say and tell others. I wasn't even married yet and feared their judgement, the 'getting pregnant before marriage' label thrown on so many women. In the many weeks that followed it took me time to come to terms and make peace with my pregnancy. While Dan was getting more and more excited, and I struggled to find acceptance with the timing completely disrupting my plans. This wasn't at all part of my plan. Getting pregnant before my wedding? I was just at the start of my career with my dreams of climbing the corporate ladder. I hadn't given much thought to becoming a mother yet, and surely not now in my mid-twenties.

Slowly I began to share the news with others and let myself get a little more excited.

At regular doctor visits and checkups, I never worried about any routine tests they did. I remember being so casual when they would bring up certain blood tests, glucose tests and others that were all part of the standard pregnancy care. I almost felt they didn't even need to do them. The timing of all of this was certainly what I had to accept, the rest of the journey was assured. It never occurred to me something could ever be wrong. The timing was a disruption in my 'life plan' so of course we are having a healthy baby just as God planned. It would be perfect. This is completely meant to be and I soon became sure of it.

"If I only would have had a sense for what was to come for us."

SOMETHING'S WRONG

SHE WAS PERFECT. RED HAIR, BRIGHT blue eyes, porcelain skin and a healthy baby. Isn't that what all parents say…. "we just want a healthy baby". Above gender, and everything else it's a healthy baby every mom prays for. Until then I had never realized the power of that statement. She weighed in just over 5lbs, and right away had this gentle calmness about her as you held her. She was like a deep breath in the ocean air.

Bringing Ali home was one of the most vulnerable days of my life. If I only would have had a sense for what was to come for us. For the first two weeks of Ali's life, she was not gaining weight. The doctors said it was quite normal and routine. What they hadn't told us was Ali had already tested twice for Cystic Fibrosis, at birth and again at her first week check-up. In Colorado she must test positive 3 times before they alert us. We had to visit the doctor daily to have her weight checked, and even with everything we tried her weight continued to decline and there was worry she wouldn't be able to thrive. Finally, the doctor told us that Ali's first tests in the hospital showed positive markers for a genetic disease called cystic fibrosis. They immediately told me there's absolutely nothing to worry about and that there are a lot of false positives, in fact 90% of positive tests don't turn out to be accurate. Still my heart dropped, but I believed them. Why had I never considered the possibility something could be wrong? She wouldn't be healthy? How could this be even possible? We were instructed she needed further testing at Children's Hospital just for safe measure to rule out any possibility of the disease. This wasn't the first time I was trying to 'rule out' something with a test. The thought terrified me.

Driving to the hospital I chose to be hopeful, and was full of anticipation to get this all over with and move forward without worry. I still didn't understand the severity of CF, looking back I don't think I wanted to. At the hospital, Ali underwent what they call a sweat test to check for the salt markers in sweat. They said that they are higher in children with cystic fibrosis as they secrete more salt in the sweat so they wrap their tiny infant wrists in material that makes them sweat, and they measure the salt levels. We were there for a few hours and I remember during the tests, the nurse kept telling me again, and again that there was nothing to worry about and it was just a routine thing that they needed to rule out. She was so sure, and I was so assured as she talked of the "young mothers so scared" having to go through this for no reason. I felt so carefree walking through the doctor's office, pushing Ali in her stroller as she slept peacefully in her tiny infant seat. Even as I said goodbye after her tests, I felt confident about the results to come. But I can clearly remember as I was leaving and making my way back to the parking garage, I got out of the elevator on the 3rd floor and saw a sign right in front of me that said "cystic fibrosis pulmonary clinic." It hit me like a ton of bricks. Inside of me I just had this feeling there was something wrong. But I ignored it, couldn't pay attention to it. If there was a way to pretend everything was fine, to deny the feeling inside something wasn't right, I mastered that on the drive home.

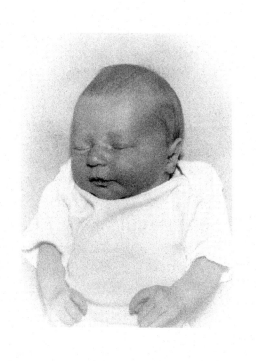

*"We didn't belong,
we were everything but perfect."*

THE CONFIRMATION

A FEW DAYS LATER, THE PHONE RANG. It was a sunny May morning and I remember the trees blooming in preparation for the summer. We had these floor to ceiling sized windows to let all of the daylight in, and as the sun shined in it lit up the room so peacefully. Ali was swinging in her swing in the corner of our living room. As I watched the swing slowly sway back and forth, it occurred to me how tiny she was. Helpless. Completely dependent on us for all of her needs, everything she needed to survive. I ran to grab the phone, "Hi Nicole, this is the nurse from the Cystic Fibrosis clinic at Children's Hospital...", the rest was a blur. I don't even know what she said. It really didn't matter. Because I knew what she was going to say. It was that doctor voice, the matter-of-fact voice with a serious, yet apologetic tone. Somehow, I managed to get off the phone keeping my composure without asking any questions. I was numb.

I don't think I moved. I didn't call anyone. I'm not even sure I was breathing in and out. I did have so many questions; Is she going to look differently? What's her life going to be like? What in the world am I supposed to do now? Is this my fault? Is this payback? Did I do something wrong?

I did remember the nurse said we needed to come down and meet with them as soon as we could. All I really wanted to do was hide, but I was desperate and needed more information. Since we had just moved and didn't have internet in our new house, I drove down to the library. In 2001 this was the fastest option for a devastated mom needing answers.

GREAT, it's story time at the library. I had just walked in and there was the circle of perfectly dressed toddlers and their happy, proud moms behind them. Happy moms because they had happy, healthy kids. Perfect kids. I hated that circle, it made me feel like an outsider. Like my baby wasn't good enough. Like I wasn't good enough. We didn't belong, we were everything but perfect.

After hiding from the circle in one of the narrow aisles I remember it smelled of old books. Ironic. I always loved books and their smell. Not today, today they were terrifying. Full of information I had to protect Ali from, information that I couldn't deny, and yet didn't want to read because once I knew how hard a life with this could be I couldn't ever unknow. I opened up a book and the very first thing I saw was that the average life expectancy for a person with cystic fibrosis is 37. Tears poured down my face and I almost collapsed as I no longer felt my legs. I had to get out of there but there was that perfect moms group, now clapping with their toddlers and singing along with the storyteller. I couldn't let them see me, I couldn't let them look at me and know we didn't belong in their circle. I ducked down carrying Ali and somehow, bravely as I was trying to be, I made it out to my car. A few minutes later pulling into our driveway I couldn't remember the drive home.

*"The breath that you just took,
that's a gift..."*

CYSTIC FIBROSIS

A COUPLE OF DAYS LATER, DAN AND I drove to children's hospital. The drive was silent and Ali slept quietly in the back. I was caught between a happy face pretending everything was fine, and defensive anger like preparation for a battle. Walking through the hospital halls you try to smile and mind your own business. Kids being pulled in wagons, exhausted parents, sickness everywhere. It was almost like an unspoken 'parents of sick kids club' agreement.... don't ask, smile like you are just fine, and pretend you are anywhere but here. Pretend it's all perfect. I really wanted to ask them, is your child ok? What is their diagnosis? Are we going to be ok? Why is this happening? But I didn't utter a word. I kept the unspoken agreement and I wondered how many of these parents were also dying inside. I didn't want to be in this club, I wanted out. My guess is they did too. It wasn't part of their plan either but no one was talking about it.

We walked into our patient room in the Pulmonary Clinic, and after we sat down the nurse left and shut the door. The door was loud and heavy. I wanted to run and scream at them nothing they would say was real. Ali was going to be fine, and we will make sure of it. I felt so angry, but at who?

Ali was curled into my body as she slept and I held her tight so tight. The room was depressing with plain white walls and a little chalkboard hung low enough for kids to draw. Someone had drawn a little stick figure I kept staring at. For a children's hospital you would think they could add a cheerful paint color to combat all the dull steel doors and counters. It resembled a jail cell. Why are we here? What are they about to tell us? Just stay focused on the stick figure Nicole and be strong. It almost felt like us against them. Why was I so angry at them before I even met them?

As I was protectively holding Ali in my arms, a whole team of people including the head doctor, nurse, dietitian and social worker entered the room. Their posture and disposition said they were all business before they even spoke. I already didn't like them. Not because they weren't going to help Ali, but because they shouldn't have to. We shouldn't even be here. This isn't supposed to happen. Don't they understand Ali isn't just some kid with some diagnosis? She was MINE. And this was not supposed to be our story!

They introduced themselves one by one. I felt outnumbered, not comforted. In a very businesslike manner the head of the CF clinic spoke of all of the things we were going to be experiencing. He started with only 50% of children with CF survive childhood, and the average life expectancy was only 37 years. How do you deliver that information to new parents just like that? No emotion. Just threw it out there for us to catch. Is there an expected way for us to receive this information? He continued to speak, but I wasn't listening. I was holding Ali tight and staring at the stick figure on the chalkboard. I didn't want to hear it anymore. No one was going to give my daughter an expectancy for life. I could feel my heart beating rapidly in my chest, and my body was stiff. I was numb. It was too much to feel. The only way to survive this appointment was to get through it and not ask questions. The pain was too much to bare.

Next the dietician. She spoke slowly, almost like she was taking pity on us. My heart started beating faster, and louder. Every time Ali ate, starting today, she would need to take enzymes to digest her food. We will start with opening capsules and sprinkling the enzymes on a spoon with applesauce before every bottle. If we missed the enzymes she could fail to thrive, and suffer awful stomach pain. Eventually as she got older she would learn to swallow the enzymes before meals. She would also need a very high fat diet since CF patients absorb less fat so we would have to make adjustments to her diet immediately.

Then the social worker. We came to find out she deals with the finances. Cystic Fibrosis can cost millions over a lifetime, and families must get their funds in order. I was supposed to go back to work after my maternity leave in about 6 weeks. Dan was working more than 12 hours a day most days, and we had just purchased our first home. How much money would we need to possibly save her life? She continued to talk about financial strains and rarely do unpaid bills go to collections. When she turns 3 she will need a therapeutic vest to help shake the bacteria and drainage out of her lungs. It would cost $16,000 and insurance doesn't cover it. I don't remember who said it, but it was recommended Ali not be in daycare to protect her from germs, colds, viruses early on. Do we get a nanny? How can we afford that? Before these last few days, I never considered being a stay-at-home-mom. I felt like I was going to throw up. This was all too much. The stick figure Nicole, look at the chalkboard. The figure was now smeared as someone had brushed against it. That's exactly how I felt. Smeared all over. Nothing was clear anymore except I was done hearing them. Done with their diagnosis and done with their pity.

"Tears poured down my face and I cried like I had never cried before in my life."

ON THE FLOOR

AS WE DROVE HOME, I WAS IN A DAZE and nothing about motherhood was turning out how I thought it would be. We found out Ali would need to visit the clinic at the hospital every 3 months for the rest of her life. Nothing about it felt normal. I wanted to picture her taking her first steps, playing preschool princess dress up and tea parties. Her graduation, learning to drive, and her wedding. Her becoming a mother and having babies of her very own. I was so angry inside, defensive, and afraid to let down my guard. Even though leaving today the doctors tried to assure us as much as they could Ali would be ok, I felt completely helpless and out of control. Dan wanted to make sure we were ok, so I told him I was going to put Ali down for a nap and get some rest myself so he could get back to work. Why was I dying on the inside, but on the outside treating this like a normal day?

After laying Ali in her crib, I lay down on our bed and so many questions were going off in my head like the firework finale on the 4th of July. Loud, fast, explosive. Our bedspread was white with tiny cheerful little red flowers all over it. I lay on my side with my head cradled in my arms; "Is she going to grow up like normal children? Will she look different? Will she fit in or be made fun of at school? Is she going to die before me? Will I have to plan her funeral?"

Why is this happening? WHY WHY WHY…. This was not the plan. This wasn't anything like I wanted it. I cried out as loud as I could without waking Ali. Tears poured down my face and I cried like I had never cried before in my life.

After what felt like days I slowly pushed myself up to check if there was blood spilling out on the bed. My heart hurt so deeply, so painfully I swore it was bleeding. I could see a large blood stain on this perfectly cheerful white bedspread. It was an invisible pool of blood, heartache that I would never forget and never look at those tiny red flowers the same after that day.

This was my moment on the floor. No not literally on the floor, but completely, entirely, wholly and fully knocked down. Warmed up, opening jog 'eye of the tiger' Rocky type entrance, in the ring all ready to rumble, and now a completely unexpected punch and you are on the floor knocked out cold and ready for the ref's 10 second countdown. That feeling of complete and utter defeat. Unable to move, unable to stand up. That moment you don't know if you can ever get back up again. If you can do this. If you have any fight left in you. If you should just curl up in a ball never to get up again. You ask yourself if anything even matters anymore. It would be so much easier to surrender. Hold up the white flag and play victim. Nothing is happening according to plan. I got a hit, a punch, and I never had a single warning or chance to prepare. The countdown starts 10... 9.... 8... I don't really care let them win.... 7.... 6.... I can't do this.... 5... there is no way I can stand up.... 4... 3... and you start to hear a little voice whisper 'you can do this'. 'You're called to do this.' Was it God? My imagination? My own mind talking? 'But you have to get up. You have to make a choice. Only you can choose' .... 2... I don't know if I can. It hurts so much. This isn't what I planned! And it was in this moment I had to choose, and no one could do it for me. Was I going to be a victim of this diagnosis or was I going to stand up, fight with everything I have, and give my daughter an amazing life? I only had two choices, and both were available. And giving up, staying on the floor would be the easiest one.

... 1.... and that's the very moment I chose to stand up and it took every single ounce of energy I had left in me. I made the commitment that my daughter was going to have an amazing life and I had no idea how, but making the decision was the first step. If I stayed on the floor, so would she. If I was a victim, she would be a victim. I had to be brave enough to stand up, for all of us.

Life had changed in a second when we had gotten the diagnosis. At the same time, life also changed again in that moment when I decided that I was going to stand up and do whatever I possibly could to fight with her, be her advocate, and give her the incredible life she deserved. There were no guarantees. But I would be brave to begin this journey with her. I would be fearless with anything coming our way that we could figure it out. I was still terrified, but I was making the choice to get off the floor and move forward anyway.

What I am sure of, we can each make that choice no matter what diagnosis comes into our lives. When we are flat on the floor, defeated, in the ring and the countdown has started. And getting up off the floor may take everything you have, but we must make a choice and only you can make it. No one can make it for you. No one will knock on the door and hand it to you. It must be you.

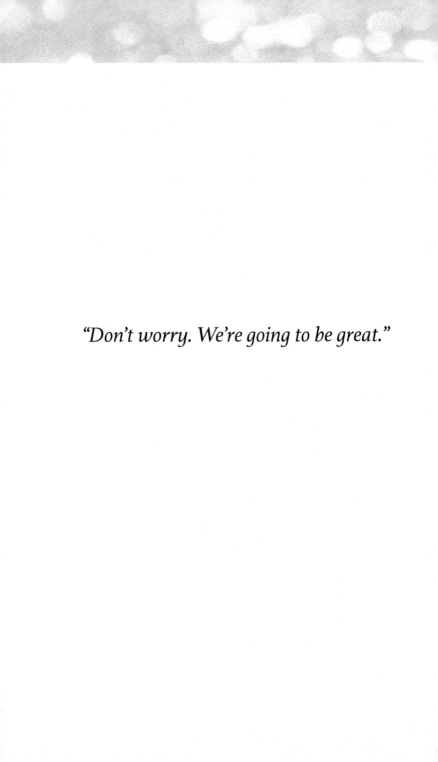

"Don't worry. We're going to be great."

SUPPORT SYSTEM

I WAS ALONE. IT ISN'T EASY TO FIND A friend that will sit with you in your pain and fully let you feel it. As a society, we assume we have to provide solutions, know the answer, stop those we love from crying or feeling hurt deeply. I wanted someone brave enough to sit with me in my pain. Fearless to enter the darkness together.

I lost a lot of my close friends in those first few months. Maybe it was circumstantial since I was in a group where I was the first to become a mother and most of my close friends were more focused on building a thriving career for their future. I wasn't able to join the happy hours, the shopping trips the places we had fun. Looking back I understand. I would cry and ask them "What if Ali dies before me?". Heavy questions for a group of girls barely entering their mid-twenties. I desperately needed a true BFF, my own 'best friend forever' willing to walk this journey with me.

It may have been then I decided my world wasn't ready for my heavy questions. They weren't ready for my vulnerability. We like to talk about the happy things, the romances, the promotions, the dreams of the future. We walk around with perfect shells, smiling faces insisting everything is great and just fine. We numb out and don't feel. But we forget when we choose numb, we also numb the joy. Not just the pain. This was a lesson I was still to learn.

My life didn't feel like happy dreams of the future. Mine was about keeping my daughter alive. And that wasn't perfect. There was nothing perfect about that. I became determined that

I was going to become the superwoman in this situation, and I was going to survive this even if I didn't talk about it with anyone. Dan and I would talk about it, but soon after Ali's diagnosis it became easier to talk about the logistics than the pain. Two people in equal pain about the same situation was not always the safest place. Perhaps we were trying to protect each other. Perhaps it was my way of protecting myself.

At some point I had made up my mind that I wasn't going to tell people about her disease, and in a lot of ways I just couldn't. I got tired of explaining what it was and what it meant. It was embarrassing for me to admit to people that I had a child that wasn't perfect because I felt like I am also judged immediately. They took pity on us. WE AREN'T PERFECT. And that would be our label. I desperately wanted to be free of all of that.

At playgroups, other moms were talking about subjects like breast feeding, sleeping routines and colic. I had all those same concerns too, but I also had much more terrifying me and often wished those were my biggest struggles. I was busy trying to empty enzyme capsules onto a teaspoon of applesauce for her to swallow before bottles just so she could digest the nutrients and hopefully absorb enough to thrive. I hid my pain and whenever it came up, I would always give my signature smile and positive voice, "Don't worry. We're going to be great."

"Sitting silently beside a friend who is hurting may be the best gift we can give."

SOMEBODY WHO UNDERSTOOD

SOON AFTER I WAS LONELY IN THE house, all day with just Ali and myself. I needed to find a mom friend. Earlier in the year we had taken a Lamaze class and there was one couple that stood out amongst a room full of expectant parents. I dug out the roster the instructor had given us and dialed her number. Voicemail. I left a message that sounded so strange saying it, like asking someone out to lunch in a new relationship.

A few weeks went by without a call back and I assumed perhaps she had found her own network to belong. I was surprised when she did finally call after being out of town, she was excited to meet. We agreed on lunch at a popular restaurant one loud enough for the babies.

As I was on my way there with Ali in the backseat, I had made up my mind that I wasn't going to tell her about Ali's Cystic Fibrosis. I was still emotionally worn out from explaining to almost everyone who asked what CF was, or hearing about their heart-breaking stories of someone they had lost. My insecurity was also taking over as I was terrified of being judged for not having a perfect healthy baby. I assumed her son was born without complication, and I didn't want to take her through my journey of pain.

We put so many expectations on ourselves. Not just as moms, as women. We are all walking around afraid of judgment, assuming our weaknesses will be labeled. Afraid to talk about the real pain because people may walk away if we are truly vulnerable. We have to do a better job for each other. To let our friends, sit in their pain without trying to fix it, or take it away.

It was the first time I sat with another new mom and felt entirely at ease since Ali was born. We weren't pretending we had it all figured out. We already knew we didn't and without much thought or hesitation I heard myself talk out loud about Ali's disease. It was a short story that I had a moment of brave to share. It was our story. I didn't get into detail, but I waited for her reaction. Her labels.

It wasn't pity. There weren't questions. There was only complete understanding. So many times, we miss that opportunity of brave to share out of fear of judgement or misunderstanding. We know once we say it, we can't take it back. It can't become unknown again. It hangs there waiting for a response, a reaction. I don't know what made me share that day, but it was a defining moment that created a completely different course of action. It was a simple moment, a simple share. A sentence of only 4 words. "Ali has Cystic Fibrosis".

Surprisingly, she said, "Oh my gosh! I know Cystic Fibrosis". In a positive tone, a collaborative tone. It was like watching a snowy forest in a Disney movie slowly turning springtime with greens and flowers. She went on, "In fact, my father-in-law's best friend started The Cystic Fibrosis Foundation in Colorado. He lost his daughter to CF and created it in her honor. We go to fundraisers, banquets, and golf tournaments...we are actively involved." The FIRST time in all these months I felt someone understood, and someone didn't think this was such a devastating situation after all.

It was an amazing light bulb to have somebody who understood. She was able to help me connect with an entire community of people in my area who really knew what we were going through. We attended formal dinners honoring the foundation and began raising money for research and a cure. Finally, I began to belong again.

Those many months before sitting in Lamaze class looking over at her I would have never known she would be a defining friend in my life. What if I hadn't been brave enough to call her, fearless enough to tell her? Fear was with me that day, she was in my pocket but I didn't let her speak. I felt free.

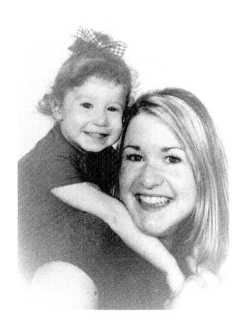

"Still a CEO, just not the way I thought it would be."

A CEO FROM HOME

BECAUSE WE WERE WARNED ABOUT medical costs and I had left my job to be with Ali, I started searching for a way to make money from home just to help us make ends meet. I remembered how helpless I felt when the doctors talked about the costs of CF and my internal commitment to make sure this wasn't an issue. Desperate, I was willing to do whatever I needed to do to help us out financially, and I never really let go of my CEO dream. I just didn't expect it would be fulfilled this way. Online through many web searches I found opportunities like home assembly and mystery shopping. Nothing seemed realistic and many options I looked into turned out to be scams asking for so much money up front. I lost money, wasted time, wanted to give up hope, but persevered. Then one day during my usual search I found an ad on the internet: a team looking for moms to work from home. Seems legit, but after so many illegitimate opportunities I was highly skeptical. So many times, I asked myself "what am I doing…how can I ever make this work?"

But I bravely filled out the form to learn more and hit the submit button. A couple of days later I received a phone call but truly I didn't really want to hear about it. Deep down I was terrified it would be another let down in my search so I almost didn't take the call. But soon as I listened to what she had to say, I heard something different. It was an opportunity to have a business, with my own hours in the wellness industry. To be part of the green movement. It was the first time I learned about the damage toxins in the home can do to our lungs, our body and immunity. This would be life changing information for Ali. Something I could truly get behind and be passionate about. And on top of it I saw the opportunity to replace my income from home, and be able to stay home with Ali. I knew it wouldn't be easy but I was committed to doing whatever it took. Desperate I said yes.

I wish I could tell you that my journey from home business to successful leader was exciting, wonderful and easy. However, as we've learned a lot doesn't always go according to plan. In fact, some of the most significant pieces of our lives often didn't happen according to our plan. But in the end, they happened perfectly. I am still a CEO of more than one business, still climbing the ladder just like I had always dreamt. It wasn't a straight road up. Not even a little. In the very beginning I lost the person I thought would be training and mentoring me, so I had to teach myself a lot. I had to become the leader I wished I'd had and I didn't have time to waste in complaining about what I didn't have. I thought about giving up when the struggles were tough, but was relentless in my commitment to Ali. I could write a book alone on the ups, downs and lessons of a homebased business. It certainly wasn't a fairy tale, but it was a commitment, a choice to making this work and do whatever it took to provide the best care and the best life for Ali.

Still a CEO, just not the way I thought it would be. But in many ways, even better.

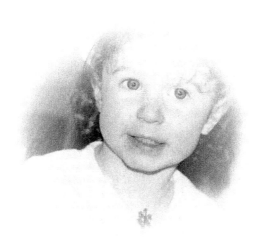

*"It's ok Ali. It's ok.
Stay still, they are almost done."*

AN INTERVENTION

ALI'S WEIGHT GAIN ISSUES WERE STILL a problem into her toddler and pre-school years. They were stressing me out day and night. I was losing sleep brainstorming of ways to help her gain weight. The doctors warned us they would need to put a feeding tube into Ali that would feed her nutrients at night so she could catch up, and have a chance thrive. We tried everything on our own to help. I added calories and fat to her drinks, cut her food into little pieces and played every feeding game known to every mom that ever lived. I played more airplane with food on a spoon than united airlines had flights every day. The struggle with CF is not only do children struggle to gain weight and absorb the fat and nutrients they need, they don't have a normal appetite like you and I and often don't feel hungry. How do you get a toddler to eat who just doesn't understand they need to eat to survive, and they aren't hungry?

I remember Ali sitting in her highchair. I had tiny pieces of pasta and cheese on her tray. I begged her to eat. I believe to this day I've said "take a bite" more than any other common phrases we say as mothers put together.

I begged her. BEGGED. Pleaded. "Please, please Ali please eat." I was getting mad. I was so mad at her. Didn't she get it? Didn't she see how desperate we were? Didn't she get the pain a feeding tube would cause her? Cause us? The complications? Didn't she get it at all? No of course she doesn't get it, she's 2.

I took it out on her, and she didn't even understand what made me so upset. This was the first day I vividly remember being so angry at her. But deep down I knew I wasn't mad at her. I was mad at all of this. ALL OF IT. I was a mom desperate to help her, desperate for answers and even more desperate to save her. I continued to plead with her. I resented the pressure I was putting around meal times, the pressure I was sure she was feeling from me. I felt shameful for the anger I put on her, but I didn't know any other way.

There was no other option. We had to start the preliminary tests for the feeding tube.

We were required to start the tests at Children's Hospital and one of the first required a tiny tube wire to be placed in her nose, down her throat and into her stomach to test for acidity, and other indicators before the stomach tube was surgically placed in. The hardest part, she would be awake. And Dan and I would have to hold her down.

As we entered the once again stale hospital room they laid Ali on the bed. I was to hold her head still, and Dan was to keep her feet still. The doctors like the parents to assist to help the children stay calm and know it is ok. I remember the bright light above Ali's head. It is so hard to be brave in these moments where our children are hurting, but I found it essential to push past my fear to be strong for her. The hardest part, she could see me and every expression I made. I had to be brave. Fearless. At least in what she saw in my eyes. Our insides can be terrified, but our outsides march forward.

As they went towards her nose she wanted to squirm. Dan had to steady her so she couldn't wiggle. I made eye contact with him for a brief second, we both looked back down. We knew the agony of the situation. I held Ali's head straight so she couldn't turn it from side to side. Her big blue eyes staring into mine. They seemed to be screaming at me. "Why are you letting them do this to me? I don't understand what is happening. This doesn't feel good."

"It's ok Ali. It's ok. Stay still they are almost done", I repeated in a strong, reassuring, nurturing tone looking straight into those terrified eyes. Dying inside, wanting to cry but not willing to let her see my fear, my tears. I was her brave.

The surgery was scheduled for the following week.

The day before the surgery I was having lunch with the chairman of the CF Foundation, and the mother who lost her daughter to CF to talk about getting more involved in awareness, and answer any questions I had. It was a hidden intervention that none of us had planned.

During lunch Ali was sitting in her high-chair happily eating her little pizza without what seemed like a care in the world.

Suddenly the women told me not to proceed with the surgery. I looked at her explaining we did all the preliminary tests and the surgery was tomorrow. Through experience they strongly believed if a child with cystic fibrosis will eat at all, then just feed them. Don't put in the tube unless they just physically can't eat. Yes, weight is going to be an ongoing struggle, but it's much better in the long run than the feeding tube. That afternoon I cancelled the surgery. Trust the information we need will be presented in the most perfect time.

"It's amazing how one little conversation can change things forever."

THE LADY FROM THE PLANE

BY THE THIRD YEAR MY BUSINESS WAS really taking off, and I retired Dan from his corporate position. I was beginning to travel a lot more and I still didn't talk too often about Cystic Fibrosis because I didn't want to feel it. Vulnerability was brave, but that meant feeling the pain. It was easier to stay busy. Busy is a way we 'numb out'. Some of us numb in other ways, binging, working out excessively, drinking….my numb of choice was staying busy. In the end, that was really what it was. It was easier not talking about it, because then I didn't have to think about it either, or let's be honest; I didn't have to hear stories of children that had passed away.

I'm one of those people when on an airplane I like to keep to myself. It's like a moment for me to breathe. I drink my yummy cup of coffee and read a magazine. This particular flight a nice older woman was sitting next to me and really wanted to talk.

Why was she trying so hard to chat with me? She was so persistent and eventually we began small talk. I told her I traveled for business and being a stay-at-home-mom this allowed me to be home with my daughter. She asked me if I could show her a picture of my daughter. I found it a little peculiar as this wasn't a question I got asked too often, this wasn't the days of smartphones where pictures are easily accessible. It meant pulling out a wallet sized picture from my purse. I stumbled through and found one to show to her and she began talking about how beautiful Ali was and her beautiful blue eyes and red hair. She asked the strangest question, she wanted to know if I chose to work from home. Then something told me to tell her. It was unlike any other conversation I had before.

The woman looked at me with the most genuine smile and said, "Oh my, I know what that is. My brother had Cystic Fibrosis."

Oh no, here comes the inevitable that I hear so often. She said 'had". Which means he's no longer here. I braced myself to hear the typical story. I really can't handle that today and I'm stuck on this plane.

She continued and said that her brother passed in his twenties. Oh no, here we go was all I could think. I got myself prepared. She must have read my hesitation.

"Oh no, you don't understand. My brother climbed every mountain there was to climb and even became a firefighter."

This wasn't the typical story I had become so used to hearing. This story had hope, a different feel. Possibility even.

She went on, "He didn't die because of cystic fibrosis. He actually died in a plane crash. He lived an amazing life. He overcame all kinds of obstacles and was able to do a lot of things even though he had the diagnosis."

Until this day, I don't know that woman's name. I don't know who she was, but she disrupted every piece of my life as a CF mama. In a single instant I realized we're not defined by our diagnosis, and only if we allow ourselves to be defined do we have to live behind that label.

Where did she come from? To me she was a walking angel, purposely placed on that plane next to me that day. What if she wasn't fearless in her conversing with me? What if she gave up as soon as she sensed I wasn't interested in talking?

Since that very day, I promised Ali never had to live behind a label for a diagnosis that she was given in her life. She would be free. A diagnosis will never define our destiny. If I had only known how important the story she told me would become one day.

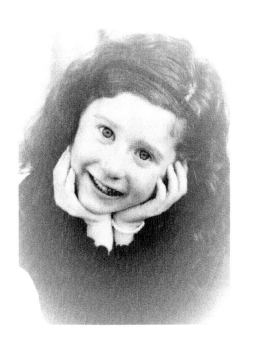

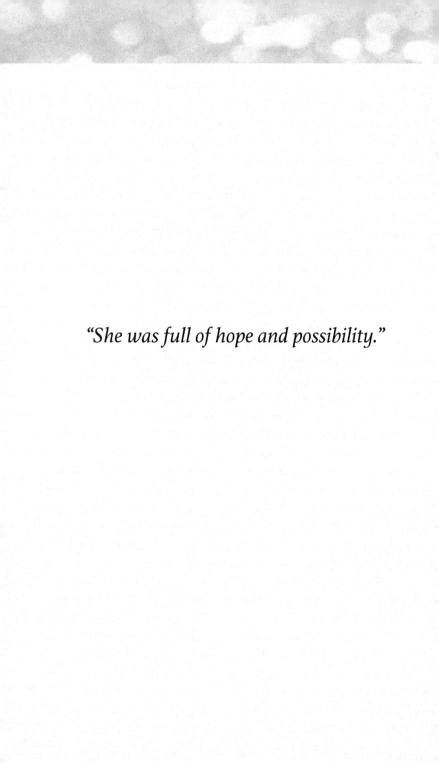

"She was full of hope and possibility."

THE 11ᵀᴴ BIRTHDAY

ONE NIGHT AFTER ALI'S 11ᵀᴴ BIRTHDAY party I was quickly trying to help her to bed, turn out the light, and collapse of exhaustion. AS I was slowly leaving her room and switching off the light, just as I was about to close her door all the way I heard her say, "Mom?". But it wasn't the normal tone she would usually use with me. It felt important. Almost desperate. I was so tired I just wanted to crawl into bed. I certainly wasn't prepared for what would come next. With the door cracked and the light off I said "yes?" hoping she couldn't sense my rushed demeanor.

"Am I going to die before you?"

Her tone was the most serious, yet more hopeful than I had ever heard. She had never asked me anything close to this before. I was floored.

I didn't think as a mom this is a question we are ever prepared for, and certainly not one often asked. But when a child considers their own mortality could be a possibility, it was the bravest question she could ever ask. And I was going to have to fearlessly answer it.

I didn't want to turn the light on because I didn't want her to see me. I knew as soon as I did those big blue eyes would be waiting to meet mine. And she desperately needed them to. I wanted to tell her absolutely not, no way. I wanted to tell her not to even think about it. To go to bed. That we could talk about it tomorrow hoping she would forget. But I didn't. If she was brave enough to ask me the question, I was going to be brave enough to answer it.

I turned her light back on and I walked over

to the bed. It felt like a million steps to get there. What in the world was I going to say? How could I not lose it? Another unfair moment I thought. What child should have to ask this, or even think about it? I wanted to tell her it wasn't fair. She drew the short stick.

Instead, I looked right into those same blue eyes that I remembered seeing when they were doing the test for the feeding tube, and I began to tell her the story of the lady from the plane.

I was able to tell her that we are all going to die, but cystic fibrosis doesn't have to determine when and how. I told her of the lady's brother who was a firefighter, and how he climbed every mountain. I told her how he lived his life full out no matter what. And then I told her about the plane crash in which took his life. I told her not any one of us is guaranteed a tomorrow. No matter what our diagnosis is. So many people live according to their diagnosis, their label, but what if none of that determines our destiny?

I was able to tell her that she can live an amazing life and absolutely nothing has to stop her. When I left her room after a long hug she looked at me differently. She was full of hope and possibility. And as I shut her door this time I couldn't help but notice in the corner her birthday balloons full of air on the ceiling just like her healthy lungs.

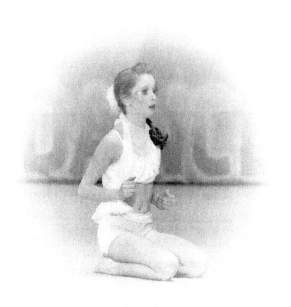

"Just because we had a diagnosis doesn't entitle us to never having another one."

BEING FREE WITH NO LIMITS

TODAY, ALI TRAINS IN COMPETITIVE dancing. She also dances at an arts school and there are times she dances for as long as 6-8 hours a day. As of now she's still at 90% lung functioning which is truly amazing for her age. She still struggles with her weight though and she takes approximately 50 pills a day to maintain her health. Her additional treatments like vest therapy which shakes the bacteria out of her lungs, and nebulizer therapy take up to an hour a day. We still visit the CF Clinic every 3 months, and as a teenager through adulthood the doctors test her every year for cystic fibrosis-related diabetes, which they tell us she will most likely develop.

Deep down I've always felt like God was telling me that it was my mission to help Ali live the best life possible. I know that no one ever promised that it was going to be easy. I remember when Ali was 5, she started competitive dancing. I remember how dedicated she was. How she worked harder than anyone I'd ever known. She showed up every day without a complaint, without an excuse, and without an expectation of an exception. I would pray just please let Ali have this one win in spite of everything she has to go through. I guess somewhere I got the idea that when life gives you a set-back or two, maybe you get a comeback somewhere else.

Well it doesn't always work that way. None of us are born with a certain amount of pain given and once we've reached the limit there isn't anymore. Just because we had a diagnosis doesn't entitle us to never having another one.

I learned Ali would have the same hardships that any other kid has. The ups, the downs, wins and losses, school struggles, and friendship troubles. Just because she has Cystic Fibrosis didn't give her a free card out of everything else. She would have to overcome those hardships just like every other kid, and she'll have to do it with Cystic Fibrosis. As a mom there were countless times I hated it. I wanted to scream it wasn't fair.

But no matter what her circumstance couldn't become an excuse. Without lowering expectations, we approached Ali's life expecting her to work at the things that she wanted just like everyone else does, and yes that may limit your time because of your disease. You may have to work harder to stay in shape, gain weight and take care of yourself but that doesn't change what you are called to do.

Today Ali wants to be a professional dancer. Medically, some would say this seems impossible, but who are we to limit her? When she talks of her dreams and shares pictures of professional dancers, I am encouraging her every step of the way.

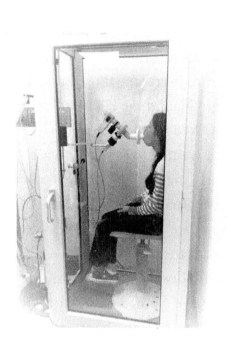

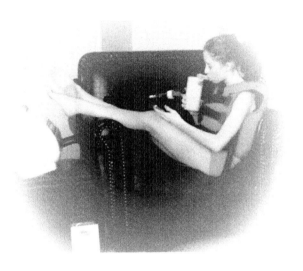

"Do not be afraid of taking big chances."

A MESSAGE FROM ALI

I WAS ABOUT NINE WHEN I FIRST BE-gan thinking more about my reality with cystic fibrosis. It was my way of life and I didn't know any other way. I've taken pills before every meal and snack and didn't know differently as long as I can remember. I've always done my treatments for breathing but about this time I really noticed my friends weren't having to do these things. I felt different. I didn't understand how serious CF was until my parents shared more with me as I got older. I was really scared about how it would affect my life. I was already having difficulties managing my time because I needed to do well in school and dance at the same time. By the 6th grade I was dancing close to 30 hours a week. I love dancing, and I hope to be a professional dancer someday. If there's one other thing that I love as much as dancing, it's travelling. I want to go to Paris and travel places outside the USA!

My mom is one of the most important people I look up to. I'm just so proud of her for who she is as a person. I'm thankful and grateful because she takes care of me, supports me, and gives me advice. I love shopping and going to lunch with my mom. She's not just a mom to me, she's a best friend.

My dad helps me keep my disease in perspective. We have a lot of fun. He helps me remember not to take everything so seriously, and enjoy life. He's the kindest person I've ever known. As I deal with my condition, I've learned more about how to take care of myself. Every morning when I wake up, I need to take my pills and eat healthy and high-fat foods.

For everyone reading this, I want you to start living your life fearlessly. Do not be afraid of taking big chances. Do not be afraid of failing. Live free by your own rules, just have fun and keep doing the things that make you happy.

I'm Ali, I'm living with a life-threatening disease called Cystic Fibrosis & I'm committed to never letting it stop me.

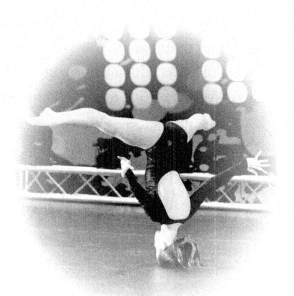

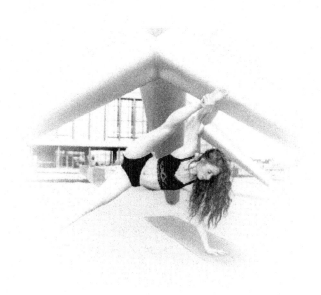

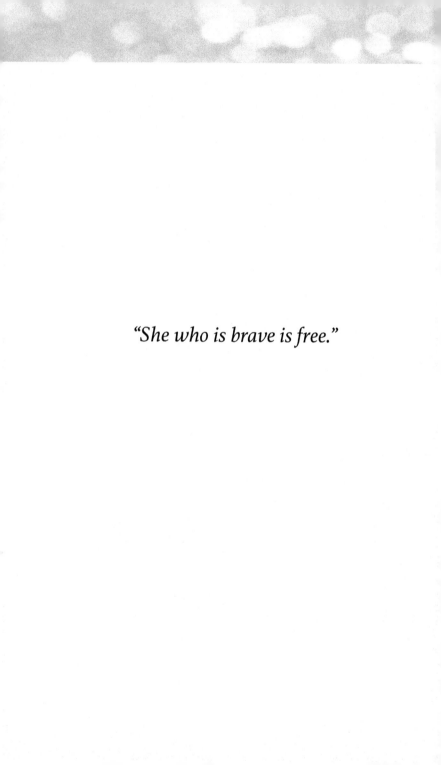

"She who is brave is free."

BEING BRAVE, FEARLESS AND FREE

I USED TO THINK THAT BEING BRAVE meant having no fear. Bravery is not being courageous without any fear. It's knowing "what is" and still being able to do the things you need to do. It's being willing to look ahead, take that first step, to have faith. It's simply doing the next right thing. Then the next without having to have it all figured out. It's believing that you do not have to live in the labels of your diagnosis, and that you can take whatever diagnosis that comes into your life and choose to get up off the floor.

I used to think that I could get to a place where I could live with no fear. But what I realized is that being fearless means being able and willing to face my fear, knowing that we're going to be okay. All of us have a diagnosis in our lives that we have to live with. It could be a disease, a label, a bankruptcy, a divorce and so on. The question I want to ask you is: Can you choose? Can you choose to live your life full out? Can we learn to be brave enough to not be perfect or numb? Can we learn to be fearless enough to look at a devastating situation and get back up off the floor so that we could live the exact way that each of us has the potential to live? I'm not going to tell you it's going to be easy, but all of us have a diagnosis that comes into our lives and knocks us down on the floor. We are called to run to our pain and not run from it. Because only there can we find our true purpose. Only then can we be truly free. Free of expectations, and free of how it was all supposed to be.

Ali is an absolutely amazing girl and she has taught me what it means to live brave, fearless and free. I've heard it said before that we must raise and celebrate the child we have, not the child we thought we would have. It's about understanding your child is exactly the person they are supposed to be. And, if we are lucky, they might just be the teacher who turns you into the person you are supposed to be.

It's all happening perfectly, all for a greater good. Find ways to be grateful and find your glimpses of joy. One of my favorites, since Ali was a little girl I've called her my ocean. People with Cystic Fibrosis often have salty skin, and with just a kiss on the cheek they taste like the salt water. I would talk about her bright, beautiful red hair like the sunset, blue eyes as pure as the water, and salty skin like the ocean air… she'll always be my ocean. And after all the ocean is one of the best places to be.

I often tell people I wouldn't change our journey. I don't know that I would take it all away even if I could. We would never be the people we have fought so hard to become. We wouldn't realize and truly understand what life really means, and that none of us have any guarantees.

I eventually made my way back to the library and into story time with that perfect mom's circle. The same one that was there when I snuck out of the library and barely made it to my car. The moms, they weren't perfect after all. They each had their own stories of being on the floor. As I watched Ali clap and sing, when she turned back and smiled at me I knew she was completely free. Free of the perfection I had expected us to be. Soon she would grow to be her own BFF. Brave, fearless and free.

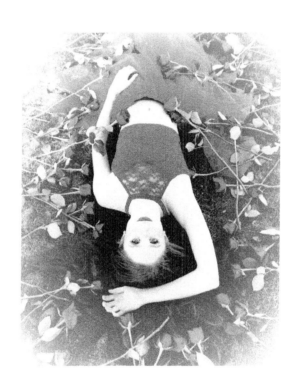

WHAT'S TO COME

BOOK TWO IN THE BFF SERIES

I was on the floor. This place, it was all too familiar to me and the memories came flooding back to me like a tidal wave. I remembered this feeling, the feeling like I can't get up and didn't know if I even wanted to. I remembered this pain. I felt it when Ali was diagnosed with cystic fibrosis. It was a pain I never wanted to feel again, and certainly never expected that I would have to. After all, how many times in our lives can we find ourselves on the floor?

It was just after midnight a few days after Christmas and I suddenly opened my eyes. No particular reason to be awake, but lying there in the middle of the night something didn't feel right. We had just hosted a joy-filled Christmas celebration at our home and the girls were fast asleep peacefully in their beds, suitcases packed, as we were leaving for Disneyland in the morning.

Before I could fall back asleep the doorbell suddenly rang and startled the house. My heart started beating so fast, who in the world would be here after midnight? I stood up quickly and cautiously walked to the doorway of the room. I could see just over the hall banister to the small window next to the front door. It was someone standing there and it looked like maybe a large flashlight sticking out of their pocket. I recognized it almost immediately to be the one the police carry with their uniform. It sounded like maybe there were others talking outside too as I could slightly make out their voices. Why in the world are the police at the door?

ACKNOWLEDGMENTS

ALI, THIS BOOK IS ABOUT A JOURNEY I would do all over again, the same way, a million more times. You awakened my purpose and gave me true meaning. I am in awe of the grace in which you handle your life. The brave, fearless, and free young woman you have become.

Isi, you are a gracious daughter and loving sister. Since the moment you were born you've been a bundle of tiny sunshine and my bond with you was instant. A smile to melt any heart.

I am so proud to be your mom. You completed me.

Dan, for bringing Ali into this world with me always handling it with such strength, and the best father Ali and Isi could ever have. We did good.

Tracy, for embracing Ali and I just as we were. Your friendship was a God given gift, in perfect timing, and left an everlasting mark on our lives.

Alexandria, for being with me that day in the office bathroom when my world was changed forever. I've never forgotten your friendship when I needed it most.

Amber, for your constant support, encouragement and always being the best cheerleader I could ever ask for.

Stacey, the business we built I am forever grateful. Thank you for being on this journey in every way.

Jenn, you've gracefully captured every picture on this journey perfectly.

Kristie, for your brand vision, patience and understanding.

Michelle, your early mentorship and support was a life line for me creating true freedom.

Lisa, for your coaching, mentoring and the direction to just get it done, and do the work.

Sean, for your creativity, support, and marketing genius.

My family, thank you for your unconditional love and support in the entire 'raising Ali' life journey. I am so blessed.

To my BFF Life friends, thank you for your ideas, stories, vulnerability and loyalty. I am so grateful to be on this journey with you.

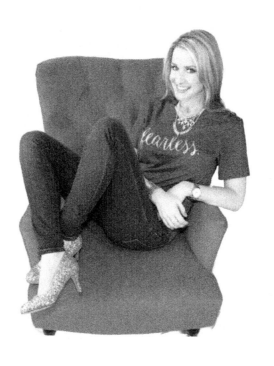

ABOUT THE AUTHOR

AT THE AGE OF TWENTY-FIVE, AFTER LEARN-
ing of her newborn daughter's diagnosis with a life-
threatening, fatal disease called Cystic Fibrosis, Nicole K.
Montez chose not to think about the limits of the situation, but the possibilities. Deciding that failure was not
an option, Nicole broke records, creating what most only
dream of: a thriving, multi-million dollar home business.
Through her elite programs she's supported and guided
professional women and gained the esteemed mentorship of some of the world's finest leaders and experts.
Nicole founded The BFF Life as a way of living, which
empowers women to live a brave, fearless and free life.
Exactly as she lives every day, equipping women with the
power to embrace and own their personal life journeys
with courage, faith and freedom. Nicole is a sought-af-
ter transformational speaker, certified success coach and
NLP, and conversation connoisseur, Nicole has lived a
story of courage and triumph that inspires live audiences
nationwide. Although her life and efforts have catapulted
her to the top, her favorite place is home, as the mother
of two amazing young ladies, Alexandra and Isabella,
who closely follow in her footsteps as talented and driven
young women. Nicole resides and thrives in Parker, CO.

CPSIA information can be obtained
at www.ICGtesting.com
Printed in the USA
LVOW03s1013201217
560367LV00002B/244/P